THE DASH DIET bible

An Easy-To-Follow Plan For Managing Hypertension And Other Cardiovascular Diseases, With Tasty Recipes

CRUE GAGE

Table of Contents

Introductory 5

CHAPTER ONE...................................9

Who Should Follow the DASH Diet?.......9

What Is Hypertension? 12

The Impact Of Diet On Hypertension ...17

CHAPTER TWO...................................24

The Principles Of The DASH Diet..........24

Meal Planning And Preparation..........30

Dash Diet Food Groups......................37

CHAPTER THREE...................................46

7-Day Meal Plan For Beginners...........46

Breakfast Recipes 56

Lunch Recipes...................................65

Dinner Recipes 74

Snacks And Desserts.........................84

CHAPTER FOUR 90

Cooking Techniques For Healthy Eating 90

Eating Out On The DASH Diet 97

Overcoming Challenges 102

Integrating Exercise With The DASH Diet
....107

Managing Other Health Conditions With
The DASH Diet 111

Conclusion...117

THE END..119

Introductory

DASH (Dietary Approaches to Stop Hypertension) is an eating regimen that is intended to assist in the treatment or prevention of hypertension. It underscores the importance of consuming foods that are high in potassium, calcium, and magnesium, which are nutrients that aid in the reduction of blood pressure. The diet is minimal in sodium, saturated fats, and added sugars.

Key components of the DASH diet include:

- **Vegetables**: Emphasizes the consumption of a variety of vegetables, including leafy greens, carrots, tomatoes, and broccoli.
- **Fruits**: Recommends several servings of fruit daily.

- **Whole Grains**: Encourages the intake of whole grains like whole wheat bread, brown rice, oatmeal, and quinoa.

- **Lean Protein**: Includes lean meats, poultry, and fish, as well as plant-based protein sources such as beans, nuts, and seeds.

- **Low-Fat Dairy**: Promotes low-fat or fat-free dairy products, such as milk, yogurt, and cheese.

- **Nuts, Seeds, and Legumes**: Suggests regular consumption of nuts, seeds, and legumes for their beneficial fats and protein.

- **Healthy Fats**: Encourages the use of healthy fats from sources like olive oil and avocados while limiting saturated fats and trans fats.

<u>Sample Daily Serving Recommendations (Based on a 2,000-Calorie Diet)</u>

- **Grains**: 6-8 servings per day
- **Vegetables**: 4-5 servings per day
- **Fruits**: 4-5 servings per day
- **Dairy**: 2-3 servings per day
- **Lean Meats, Poultry, and Fish**: 6 or fewer servings (1 oz each) per day
- **Nuts, Seeds, and Legumes**: 4-5 servings per week
- **Fats and Oils**: 2-3 servings per day
- **Sweets**: 5 or fewer servings per week

<u>Benefits of the DASH Diet:</u>

- **Blood Pressure Reduction**: Proven to lower blood pressure in both hypertensive and normotensive individuals.

- **Weight Loss**: Can help with weight loss if combined with calorie restriction and increased physical activity.
- **Overall Health**: Promotes heart health and reduces the risk of cardiovascular diseases, stroke, and certain types of cancer.

The DASH diet is flexible and balanced, making it a sustainable long-term eating plan for many people.

CHAPTER ONE
Who Should Follow the DASH Diet?

The DASH diet is beneficial for a wide range of people, particularly those concerned with maintaining or improving cardiovascular health. Here are some specific groups who may particularly benefit from following the DASH diet:

• Individuals with High Blood Pressure (Hypertension): The DASH diet is specifically designed to lower blood pressure and has been shown to be effective in doing so.

• Those at Risk of Developing Hypertension: People with prehypertension or a family history of high blood pressure can benefit from following the DASH diet to help prevent the onset of hypertension.

• **People with Heart Disease**: Since the diet promotes heart-healthy eating habits, it can help reduce the risk of heart disease and improve overall cardiovascular health.

• **Individuals with Diabetes**: The DASH diet helps in managing blood sugar levels due to its emphasis on whole grains, fruits, vegetables, and lean proteins while limiting sugar and refined carbohydrates.

• **People Looking to Lose Weight**: While not specifically a weight loss diet, the DASH diet can support weight loss efforts due to its emphasis on nutrient-dense, low-calorie foods.

• **Those with High Cholesterol**: The diet's focus on reducing saturated fats and cholesterol can help lower LDL (bad) cholesterol levels.

• **Anyone Seeking a Balanced, Healthy Diet**: The DASH diet is well-rounded and emphasizes a variety of foods, making it a good option for anyone looking to improve their overall nutrition and health.

• **Individuals with Chronic Kidney Disease**: The diet's focus on reducing sodium intake can be beneficial for kidney health.

While the DASH diet is generally considered safe and healthy for most people, it's always a good idea to consult with a healthcare provider before making significant dietary changes, especially for those with specific health conditions or dietary needs.

What Is Hypertension?

Hypertension, commonly known as high blood pressure, is a medical condition where the force of the blood against the artery walls is consistently too high. This can lead to various health problems, such as heart disease, stroke, and kidney disease. Blood pressure is measured in millimeters of mercury (mm Hg) and is recorded with two numbers: systolic pressure (the top number) and diastolic pressure (the bottom number).

Blood Pressure Categories:

- **Normal Blood Pressure**: Systolic less than 120 mm Hg and diastolic less than 80 mm Hg.
- **Elevated Blood Pressure**: Systolic between 120-129 mm Hg and diastolic less than 80 mm Hg.

- **Hypertension Stage 1**: Systolic between 130-139 mm Hg or diastolic between 80-89 mm Hg.

- **Hypertension Stage 2**: Systolic 140 mm Hg or higher or diastolic 90 mm Hg or higher.

- **Hypertensive Crisis**: Systolic higher than 180 mm Hg and/or diastolic higher than 120 mm Hg, which requires immediate medical attention.

Causes of Hypertension:

- **Genetics**: Family history can play a role.

- **Unhealthy Diet**: High in salt, saturated fats, and cholesterol.

- **Physical Inactivity**: Lack of exercise contributes to high blood pressure.

- **Obesity**: Excess weight increases the strain on the heart.
- **Smoking**: Tobacco use raises blood pressure.
- **Excessive Alcohol Consumption**: Can lead to hypertension.
- **Stress**: Chronic stress may contribute to high blood pressure.
- **Age**: Blood pressure tends to increase with age.
- **Chronic Conditions**: Such as kidney disease, diabetes, and sleep apnea.

<u>Symptoms of Hypertension:</u>

Hypertension is often called a "silent killer" because it usually has no noticeable symptoms.

<u>**However, in severe cases or hypertensive crisis, symptoms can include:**</u>

- Severe headaches
- Shortness of breath
- Nosebleeds
- Severe anxiety

<u>**Complications of Hypertension:**</u>

- If left untreated, hypertension can lead to:
- Heart attack or stroke
- Aneurysm
- Heart failure
- Weakened and narrowed blood vessels in the kidneys
- Thickened, narrowed, or torn blood vessels in the eyes
- Metabolic syndrome
- Cognitive decline and dementia

Management and Treatment

Lifestyle Changes:

- Healthy diet (like the DASH diet)
- Regular physical activity
- Maintaining a healthy weight
- Reducing salt intake
- Limiting alcohol consumption
- Quitting smoking
- Managing stress

Medications: Various medications can help control blood pressure, including diuretics, ACE inhibitors, angiotensin II receptor blockers (ARBs), calcium channel blockers, and beta-blockers.

Regular Monitoring: Regular check-ups and monitoring blood pressure at home can help manage and control hypertension effectively.

Early detection and management of hypertension are crucial to reduce the risk of serious health complications.

The Impact Of Diet On Hypertension

Diet plays a crucial role in the management and prevention of hypertension. Here are some specific ways in which diet impacts blood pressure:

<u>Sodium Intake:</u>

• **High Sodium**: Excessive sodium intake is a major contributor to high blood pressure. Sodium causes the body to retain water, which increases blood volume and, consequently, blood pressure.

• **Reducing Sodium**: Lowering sodium intake can significantly reduce blood pressure, especially in people who are salt-sensitive. The American Heart Association recommends consuming no more than 2,300 milligrams of sodium per day, with an ideal limit of 1,500 milligrams for most adults.

Potassium, Calcium, and Magnesium:

• **Potassium**: Helps balance the amount of sodium in cells, which can reduce blood pressure. Foods rich in potassium include bananas, potatoes, spinach, and beans.

• **Calcium**: Essential for vascular contraction and vasodilation (the tightening and relaxation of blood vessels). Low-fat dairy products, leafy greens, and fortified foods are good sources of calcium.

• **Magnesium**: Helps regulate blood pressure. Whole grains, nuts, seeds, and green leafy vegetables are good sources of magnesium.

Fruits and Vegetables:

• **Rich in Nutrients**: Fruits and vegetables are high in vitamins, minerals, and fiber but low in calories and sodium. They provide potassium, magnesium, and antioxidants, which help lower blood pressure.

• **DASH Diet**: Emphasizes the consumption of a variety of fruits and vegetables, contributing to its effectiveness in lowering blood pressure.

Whole Grains:

• **Fiber and Nutrients**: Whole grains are rich in fiber and essential nutrients that can help manage blood pressure. Foods like whole wheat bread, brown rice, and oatmeal are beneficial.

Healthy Fats:

• **Unsaturated Fats**: Found in olive oil, avocados, nuts, and seeds, can help reduce blood pressure. Omega-3 fatty acids, found in fatty fish like salmon and mackerel, also have heart health benefits.

• **Saturated and Trans Fats**: Should be limited as they can contribute to high blood pressure and cardiovascular disease.

<u>Lean Proteins:</u>

• **Plant-Based Proteins**: Beans, lentils, and soy products are good sources of protein that can help manage blood pressure.

• **Lean Animal Proteins**: Poultry, fish, and low-fat dairy products are preferred over red and processed meats.

<u>Reducing Added Sugars and Refined Carbohydrates:</u>

• **Added Sugars**: High consumption of sugary foods and drinks is linked to increased blood pressure.

• **Refined Carbohydrates**: Such as white bread and sugary cereals can cause spikes in blood sugar and insulin, leading to higher blood pressure.

<u>Alcohol Intake:</u>

• **Moderation**: Excessive alcohol consumption can raise blood pressure. It's recommended that men limit alcohol to two drinks per day and women to one drink per day.

<u>Caffeine:</u>

• **Temporary Increase**: Caffeine can cause a short-term spike in blood pressure. However, for most people, regular caffeine consumption does not have a significant long-term impact on blood pressure.

A balanced diet that is low in sodium and rich in potassium, calcium, and magnesium can help prevent and manage hypertension. Reducing the intake of unhealthy fats, added sugars, and refined carbohydrates, while increasing the consumption of fruits, vegetables, whole grains, and lean proteins, is essential for maintaining healthy blood pressure levels.

CHAPTER TWO
The Principles Of The DASH Diet

The DASH (Dietary Approaches to Stop Hypertension) diet is built on specific principles aimed at promoting cardiovascular health and lowering blood pressure. Here are the key principles:

1. Rich in Fruits and Vegetables:

- **Servings**: 4-5 servings of each per day.
- **Benefits**: These foods are high in potassium, magnesium, and fiber, which are essential for controlling blood pressure.

2. Emphasis on Whole Grains:

- **Servings**: 6-8 servings per day.
- **Benefits**: Whole grains are high in fiber and nutrients, promoting

heart health and helping to manage blood pressure.

3. Lean Proteins:

- **Sources**: Lean meats, poultry, fish, and plant-based proteins like beans, nuts, and seeds.
- **Servings**: 6 or fewer servings of lean meat per day (1 oz each), 4-5 servings of nuts, seeds, and legumes per week.
- **Benefits**: Provides essential nutrients while limiting saturated fats.

4. Low-Fat or Fat-Free Dairy:

- **Servings**: 2-3 servings per day.
- **Benefits**: Provides calcium and vitamin D without the added

saturated fat found in full-fat dairy products.

5. Healthy Fats:

- **Sources**: Unsaturated fats from oils like olive oil, nuts, seeds, and avocados.
- **Servings**: 2-3 servings per day.
- **Benefits**: Supports heart health by reducing bad cholesterol levels.

6. Low in Sodium:

- **Limit**: Ideally less than 1,500 mg per day; no more than 2,300 mg per day.
- **Benefits**: Reducing sodium intake helps lower blood pressure and reduces the risk of heart disease and stroke.

7. Limited Sweets and Added Sugars:

- **Servings**: 5 or fewer servings per week.
- **Benefits**: Helps maintain healthy blood pressure and weight by reducing empty calorie intake.

8. Limited Red and Processed Meats:

- **Recommendation**: Substitute with lean meats, fish, or plant-based proteins.
- **Benefits**: Reduces intake of saturated fats and cholesterol.

9. Increased Potassium, Magnesium, and Calcium:

- **Sources**: Through a diet rich in fruits, vegetables, low-fat dairy, nuts, seeds, and whole grains.

- **Benefits**: These minerals are crucial for blood pressure regulation.

10. Moderation in Alcohol Consumption:

- **Limit**: Men should have no more than two drinks per day, and women no more than one.
- **Benefits**: Helps prevent the rise in blood pressure associated with excessive alcohol intake.

<u>Sample Daily Plan (2,000-Calorie Diet):</u>

- **Grains**: 6-8 servings (e.g., whole grain bread, brown rice, oatmeal)
- **Vegetables**: 4-5 servings (e.g., leafy greens, carrots, broccoli)
- **Fruits**: 4-5 servings (e.g., apples, oranges, berries)

- **Dairy**: 2-3 servings (e.g., low-fat milk, yogurt, cheese)
- **Lean Meats, Poultry, and Fish**: 6 or fewer servings (1 oz each)
- **Nuts, Seeds, and Legumes**: 4-5 servings per week
- **Fats and Oils**: 2-3 servings (e.g., olive oil, avocado)
- **Sweets**: 5 or fewer servings per week (e.g., small amounts of sugar, jelly, or candy)

The DASH diet is flexible and can be adapted to meet individual dietary needs and preferences, making it a practical approach for improving health and managing blood pressure.

Meal Planning And Preparation

Meal planning and preparation are key to successfully following the DASH diet. Here are some tips and strategies to help you get started:

Steps for Effective Meal Planning

Assess Your Needs:

- Determine your daily caloric needs based on your age, sex, activity level, and health goals.
- Plan for a variety of foods to ensure you get a balance of nutrients.

Create a Weekly Meal Plan:

- Outline your meals and snacks for the week, focusing on the DASH diet guidelines.

- Include plenty of fruits, vegetables, whole grains, lean proteins, and low-fat dairy.

Make a Shopping List:

- Based on your meal plan, list all the ingredients you'll need.
- Stick to your list to avoid impulse buys and ensure you have everything you need for healthy meals.

Prep in Advance:

- Set aside time to wash, chop, and store vegetables and fruits.
- Cook large batches of grains, beans, and lean proteins that can be used throughout the week.

- Portion out snacks like nuts, seeds, and cut-up veggies to have on hand.

Sample Meal Plan for One Day (2,000-Calorie Diet):

Breakfast:

- **Oatmeal**: 1 cup cooked oats topped with fresh berries and a handful of nuts
- **Low-Fat Milk**: 1 cup
- **Orange**: 1 medium

Mid-Morning Snack:

- **Greek Yogurt**: 1 cup low-fat with a drizzle of honey
- **Apple**: 1 medium

Lunch

- **Grilled Chicken Salad**: Mixed greens with grilled chicken breast, cherry tomatoes, cucumbers, bell peppers, and a vinaigrette dressing
- **Whole Grain Roll**: 1 small
- **Low-Fat Cheese**: 1 ounce

Afternoon Snack:

- **Carrot Sticks**: 1 cup
- **Hummus**: 1/4 cup

Dinner:

- **Baked Salmon**: 4 ounces with a squeeze of lemon
- **Quinoa**: 1/2 cup cooked
- **Steamed Broccoli**: 1 cup
- **Side Salad**: Mixed greens with olive oil and balsamic vinegar

Evening Snack

- **Air-Popped Popcorn**: 3 cups
- **Almonds**: 1/4 cup

Meal Prep Tips

- **Batch Cooking**: Prepare large quantities of grains, lean proteins, and legumes that can be used in various dishes throughout the week.
- **Pre-Portioning**: Store meals in individual containers for easy grab-and-go options.
- **Utilize Leftovers**: Repurpose leftovers into new meals (e.g., grilled chicken from dinner can be used in a salad for lunch).
- **Freezing**: Freeze extra portions of soups, stews, and casseroles for quick meals later on.

- **Healthy Snacks**: Keep healthy snacks like fruits, veggies, yogurt, and nuts readily available.

Shopping Tips

- **Perimeter Shopping**: Focus on the outer aisles of the grocery store where fresh produce, meats, and dairy are usually found.
- **Read Labels**: Check nutrition labels for sodium, added sugars, and unhealthy fats.
- **Seasonal Produce**: Buy seasonal fruits and vegetables for better taste and lower cost.
- **Frozen and Canned Options**: Choose no-salt-added canned vegetables and fruits packed in water or their own juice. Frozen fruits and vegetables without

added sauces or sugars are also good options.

<u>Sample Grocery List</u>

Fruits and Vegetables:

- Apples, oranges, berries
- Leafy greens (spinach, kale, lettuce)
- Carrots, bell peppers, cucumbers
- Broccoli, cauliflower
- Sweet potatoes, tomatoes

Grains

- Whole grain bread, brown rice, quinoa, oats

Proteins

- Chicken breast, salmon, lean beef
- Eggs
- Beans, lentils, chickpeas

- Nuts and seeds

Dairy

- Low-fat milk, yogurt, cheese

Others

- Olive oil, vinegar, spices, herbs
- Hummus
- Whole grain roll

By planning meals and preparing ingredients ahead of time, you can make following the DASH diet easier and more convenient, ensuring you stick to the dietary guidelines and enjoy a variety of nutritious meals.

Dash Diet Food Groups

The DASH (Dietary Approaches to Stop Hypertension) diet emphasizes a variety of food groups to provide essential nutrients and promote overall health. Here is a detailed look at the food groups included in the DASH diet, along with recommended servings and examples:

1. Grains:

- **Servings**: 6-8 servings per day
- **Benefits**: Whole grains are a great source of energy and provide essential nutrients such as fiber, B vitamins, and minerals.
- **Examples**: Whole wheat bread, brown rice, quinoa, oatmeal, whole grain pasta, barley

2. Vegetables:

- **Servings**: 4-5 servings per day
- **Benefits**: Vegetables are high in vitamins, minerals, fiber, and antioxidants, which help lower

blood pressure and improve overall health.

- **Examples**: Leafy greens (spinach, kale), broccoli, carrots, bell peppers, tomatoes, squash, sweet potatoes

3. Fruits:

- **Servings**: 4-5 servings per day
- **Benefits**: Fruits are rich in fiber, vitamins, especially vitamin C and potassium, which helps in regulating blood pressure.
- **Examples**: Apples, oranges, bananas, berries, grapes, melons, peaches, pears

4. Dairy:

- **Servings**: 2-3 servings per day

- **Benefits**: Low-fat or fat-free dairy products provide calcium, vitamin D, and protein without the added saturated fat.

- **Examples**: Low-fat milk, yogurt, cheese

5. Lean Meats, Poultry, and Fish:

- **Servings**: 6 or fewer servings per day (1 oz each)

- **Benefits**: These protein sources are important for muscle maintenance and provide essential nutrients like iron and zinc while being low in saturated fat.

- **Examples**: Skinless chicken breast, turkey, fish (especially fatty fish like salmon and mackerel), lean cuts of beef and pork

6. Nuts, Seeds, and Legumes:

- **Servings**: 4-5 servings per week
- **Benefits**: These foods are excellent sources of protein, magnesium, potassium, and fiber. They also contain healthy fats that are beneficial for heart health.
- **Examples**: Almonds, walnuts, sunflower seeds, flaxseeds, lentils, chickpeas, black beans

7. Fats and Oils:

- **Servings**: 2-3 servings per day
- **Benefits**: Healthy fats are crucial for the absorption of fat-soluble vitamins and provide essential fatty acids that support heart health.
- **Examples**: Olive oil, canola oil, avocado, nuts, seeds

8. Sweets and Added Sugars

- **Servings**: 5 or fewer servings per week

- **Benefits**: Limiting sweets helps control calorie intake and reduces the risk of weight gain, which can affect blood pressure.

- **Examples**: Sugar, jelly, candy, sweetened beverages, desserts

Daily Caloric Intake and Portion Sizes:

The number of servings you need from each food group depends on your daily calorie requirements. Here is a guideline based on a 2,000-calorie diet:

- **Grains**: 1 slice of bread, 1/2 cup cooked rice or pasta, 1 oz dry cereal

- **Vegetables**: 1 cup raw leafy vegetables, 1/2 cup cooked vegetables, 1/2 cup vegetable juice

- **Fruits**: 1 medium fruit, 1/2 cup fresh, frozen, or canned fruit, 1/2 cup fruit juice

- **Dairy**: 1 cup milk or yogurt, 1.5 oz cheese

- **Lean Meats, Poultry, Fish**: 1 oz cooked meat, poultry, or fish

- **Nuts, Seeds, Legumes**: 1/3 cup or 1.5 oz nuts, 2 tablespoons peanut butter, 1/2 cup cooked beans or peas

- **Fats and Oils**: 1 teaspoon soft margarine, 1 teaspoon vegetable oil, 1 tablespoon mayonnaise, 2 tablespoons salad dressing

- **Sweets**: 1 tablespoon sugar, jelly, or jam, 1/2 cup sorbet, 1 cup lemonade

Tips for Incorporating DASH Diet Foods:

- **Gradual Changes**: Introduce new foods and increase servings gradually to adapt to the diet without feeling overwhelmed.

- **Diverse Choices**: Vary your food choices within each group to ensure a wide range of nutrients.

- **Healthy Snacks**: Opt for fruits, vegetables, nuts, and low-fat dairy for snacks.

- **Balanced Meals**: Include multiple food groups in each meal to maintain a balanced diet.

- **Reduce Sodium**: Choose fresh or frozen vegetables over canned ones, use herbs and spices for seasoning, and check labels for low-sodium options.

By following these guidelines and focusing on these food groups, the DASH diet can help manage blood pressure and promote overall health.

CHAPTER THREE
7-Day Meal Plan For Beginners

Creating a 7-day meal plan for beginners on the DASH diet involves incorporating a variety of foods from the different food groups while keeping meals simple and easy to prepare. Here's a sample 7-day meal plan to get you started:

<u>Day 1</u>

Breakfast:

- Oatmeal with fresh berries and a handful of nuts
- Low-fat milk

Mid-Morning Snack:

- Apple slices with a tablespoon of peanut butter

Lunch:

- Grilled chicken salad with mixed greens, cherry tomatoes, cucumbers, and a vinaigrette dressing
- Whole grain roll

Afternoon Snack:

- Carrot sticks with hummus

Dinner:

- Baked salmon with lemon and herbs
- Quinoa
- Steamed broccoli

Evening Snack:

- Air-popped popcorn

Day 2

Breakfast:

- Greek yogurt with honey and a banana

Mid-Morning Snack:

- A handful of almonds

Lunch:

- Whole grain turkey sandwich with lettuce, tomato, and mustard
- Side of baby carrots

Afternoon Snack:

- Low-fat cheese and whole grain crackers

Dinner:

- Stir-fried tofu with mixed vegetables (broccoli, bell peppers, snap peas) and brown rice

Evening Snack:

- Fresh fruit salad

Day 3

Breakfast:

- Whole grain toast with avocado and a boiled egg

Mid-Morning Snack:

- Orange

Lunch:

- Lentil soup with a side of mixed greens salad

Afternoon Snack:

- Celery sticks with almond butter

Dinner:

- Grilled shrimp with a side of couscous
- Steamed asparagus

Evening Snack:

- Low-fat yogurt with a sprinkle of flaxseeds

<u>Day 4</u>

Breakfast:

- Smoothie with spinach, banana, berries, and low-fat milk

Mid-Morning Snack:

- Handful of walnuts

Lunch:

- Quinoa salad with black beans, corn, cherry tomatoes, and a lime vinaigrette

Afternoon Snack:

- Sliced bell peppers with guacamole

Dinner:

- Baked chicken breast with a side of wild rice
- Roasted Brussels sprouts

Evening Snack:

- Pear slices

<u>**Day 5**</u>

Breakfast:

- Whole grain cereal with low-fat milk and sliced strawberries

Mid-Morning Snack:

- Low-fat string cheese

Lunch:

- Tuna salad (tuna, mixed greens, cucumbers, cherry tomatoes, olives) with whole grain crackers

Afternoon Snack:

- Fresh fruit (apple or pear)

Dinner:

- Turkey chili with kidney beans and a side of whole grain cornbread

- Mixed greens salad

Evening Snack:

- Handful of mixed nuts

<u>Day 6</u>

Breakfast:

- Whole grain pancakes with fresh blueberries and a dollop of low-fat yogurt

Mid-Morning Snack:

- Grapes

Lunch:

- Chickpea and vegetable wrap with whole grain tortilla

Afternoon Snack:

- Sliced cucumbers with tzatziki

Dinner:

- Baked cod with a side of barley
- Sautéed spinach

Evening Snack:

- Fresh mango slices

<u>**Day 7**</u>

Breakfast:

- Scrambled eggs with spinach and whole grain toast

Mid-Morning Snack:

- Banana

Lunch:

- Chicken and vegetable stir-fry with brown rice

Afternoon Snack:

- Low-fat yogurt with a handful of granola

Dinner:

- Grilled salmon with a side of quinoa and steamed green beans

Evening Snack:

- Mixed berries

<u>Tips for Success:</u>

- **Meal Prep**: Prepare and portion out ingredients ahead of time to make cooking easier during the week.
- **Variety**: Mix and match meals and snacks to keep things interesting.
- **Hydration**: Drink plenty of water throughout the day.

- **Spices and Herbs**: Use spices and herbs to enhance the flavor of your dishes without adding extra sodium.

- **Portion Control**: Pay attention to portion sizes to avoid overeating.

By following this 7-day meal plan, beginners can easily get started on the DASH diet and enjoy a variety of delicious and healthy meals.

Breakfast Recipes

Here are some easy and delicious breakfast recipes that align with the DASH diet principles:

1. Oatmeal with Berries and Nuts

Ingredients:

- 1 cup rolled oats

- 2 cups water or low-fat milk

- 1/2 cup mixed berries (strawberries, blueberries, raspberries)
- 1 tablespoon nuts (almonds, walnuts, or pecans)
- 1 teaspoon honey or maple syrup (optional)

Instructions:

- In a saucepan, bring the water or milk to a boil.
- Add the oats and reduce the heat to a simmer.
- Cook for about 5 minutes, stirring occasionally until the oats are soft.
- Top with mixed berries, nuts, and a drizzle of honey or maple syrup if desired.

2. Greek Yogurt Parfait:

Ingredients:

- 1 cup low-fat Greek yogurt
- 1/2 cup granola (choose a low-sugar option)
- 1/2 cup fresh fruit (such as berries, sliced banana, or chopped apple)
- 1 tablespoon chia seeds or flaxseeds (optional)

Instructions:

- In a glass or bowl, layer the yogurt, granola, and fresh fruit.
- Sprinkle chia seeds or flaxseeds on top for added fiber and nutrients.
- Repeat layers if desired and serve immediately.

3. Avocado Toast with Egg:

Ingredients:

- 1 slice whole grain bread
- 1/2 avocado
- 1 egg (poached, scrambled, or boiled)
- Salt and pepper to taste
- Optional toppings: cherry tomatoes, red pepper flakes, or a squeeze of lemon juice

Instructions:

- Toast the slice of whole grain bread until golden brown.
- While the bread is toasting, prepare the egg to your liking.
- Mash the avocado in a small bowl and season with salt and pepper.

- Spread the mashed avocado on the toasted bread.
- Top with the cooked egg and any additional toppings you prefer.

4. Smoothie with Spinach, Banana, and Berries:

Ingredients:

- 1 cup fresh spinach
- 1 banana
- 1/2 cup mixed berries (fresh or frozen)
- 1 cup low-fat milk or unsweetened almond milk
- 1 tablespoon chia seeds (optional)

Instructions:

- Place all ingredients in a blender.

- Blend until smooth, adding more milk if needed to reach your desired consistency.
- Pour into a glass and enjoy immediately.

5. Whole Grain Pancakes

Ingredients:

- 1 cup whole wheat flour
- 1 tablespoon baking powder
- 1/4 teaspoon salt
- 1 cup low-fat milk
- 1 egg
- 2 tablespoons vegetable oil or melted butter
- 1 tablespoon honey or maple syrup (optional)
- Fresh berries or sliced fruit for topping

Instructions:

- In a large bowl, whisk together the whole wheat flour, baking powder, and salt.
- In another bowl, whisk together the milk, egg, oil or butter, and honey or maple syrup.
- Pour the wet ingredients into the dry ingredients and stir until just combined (do not overmix).
- Heat a non-stick skillet or griddle over medium heat and lightly grease with oil or cooking spray.
- Pour 1/4 cup of batter onto the skillet for each pancake.
- Cook until bubbles form on the surface, then flip and cook until golden brown on the other side.
- Serve with fresh berries or sliced fruit on top.

6. Scrambled Eggs with Spinach and Tomatoes:

Ingredients:

- 2 eggs
- 1/4 cup low-fat milk
- 1/2 cup fresh spinach, chopped
- 1/4 cup cherry tomatoes, halved
- Salt and pepper to taste
- 1 teaspoon olive oil

Instructions:

- In a bowl, whisk together the eggs and milk, and season with salt and pepper.
- Heat the olive oil in a non-stick skillet over medium heat.
- Add the spinach and tomatoes, and cook until the spinach is wilted.

- Pour the egg mixture into the skillet and cook, stirring gently, until the eggs are set.
- Serve immediately with whole grain toast if desired.

7. Cottage Cheese with Fruit and Nuts:

Ingredients:

- 1 cup low-fat cottage cheese
- 1/2 cup fresh fruit (such as pineapple, peaches, or berries)
- 1 tablespoon chopped nuts (such as almonds or walnuts)
- 1 teaspoon honey (optional)

Instructions:

- Place the cottage cheese in a bowl.
- Top with fresh fruit and chopped nuts.

- Drizzle with honey if desired and serve.

These recipes provide a good balance of nutrients and flavors to help you start your day on the right foot while adhering to the DASH diet principles.

Lunch Recipes

Here are some easy and nutritious lunch recipes that fit well within the DASH diet guidelines:

1. Quinoa Salad with Black Beans and Avocado:

Ingredients:

- 1 cup cooked quinoa
- 1 can (15 oz) black beans, rinsed and drained
- 1 avocado, diced
- 1 cup cherry tomatoes, halved

- 1/4 cup red onion, diced
- Juice of 1 lime
- Salt and pepper to taste
- Fresh cilantro (optional)

Instructions:

- In a large bowl, combine the quinoa, black beans, avocado, cherry tomatoes, and red onion.
- Drizzle with lime juice and season with salt and pepper.
- Toss gently to combine and garnish with cilantro if desired.

2. Turkey and Spinach Wrap:

Ingredients:

- 1 whole grain tortilla
- 4 oz sliced turkey breast (low sodium)
- 1/2 cup fresh spinach

* 1/4 cup sliced cucumber

* 1/4 cup shredded carrots

* 1 tablespoon hummus or mustard

Instructions:

* Spread hummus or mustard over the tortilla.

* Layer the turkey, spinach, cucumber, and carrots on top.

* Roll the tortilla tightly and slice in half to serve.

3. Lentil Soup:

Ingredients:

* 1 cup dried lentils, rinsed

* 1 medium onion, chopped

* 2 carrots, diced

* 2 celery stalks, diced

* 2 cloves garlic, minced

- 6 cups vegetable broth (low sodium)
- 1 teaspoon cumin
- Salt and pepper to taste
- Fresh parsley for garnish (optional)

Instructions:

- In a large pot, sauté onion, carrots, celery, and garlic over medium heat until softened.
- Add lentils, vegetable broth, cumin, salt, and pepper.
- Bring to a boil, then reduce heat and simmer for 30-40 minutes, until lentils are tender.
- Garnish with fresh parsley before serving.

4. Chickpea Salad:

Ingredients:

- 1 can (15 oz) chickpeas, rinsed and drained
- 1 cup diced cucumber
- 1 cup cherry tomatoes, halved
- 1/4 cup red onion, diced
- Juice of 1 lemon
- 1 tablespoon olive oil
- Salt and pepper to taste
- Fresh parsley or basil (optional)

Instructions:

- In a bowl, combine chickpeas, cucumber, cherry tomatoes, and red onion.
- Drizzle with lemon juice and olive oil; season with salt and pepper.

- Toss gently and garnish with fresh herbs if desired.

5. Vegetable Stir-Fry:

Ingredients:

- 1 cup mixed vegetables (broccoli, bell peppers, snap peas, carrots)
- 1/2 cup firm tofu, cubed (or chicken/shrimp for non-vegetarian)
- 2 tablespoons low-sodium soy sauce
- 1 teaspoon sesame oil (optional)
- Cooked brown rice or quinoa for serving

Instructions:

- Heat a non-stick skillet or wok over medium-high heat.

- Add the tofu (or protein of choice) and cook until golden brown.
- Add mixed vegetables and stir-fry for about 5-7 minutes until tender-crisp.
- Stir in soy sauce and sesame oil, cooking for an additional 2 minutes.
- Serve over brown rice or quinoa.

6. Grilled Chicken Salad:

Ingredients:

- 4 oz grilled chicken breast, sliced
- Mixed greens (spinach, arugula, romaine)
- 1/2 cup cherry tomatoes, halved
- 1/4 cup cucumber, sliced
- 1/4 cup shredded carrots
- Balsamic vinaigrette or lemon juice for dressing

Instructions:

- In a large bowl, combine mixed greens, cherry tomatoes, cucumber, and carrots.
- Top with sliced grilled chicken.
- Drizzle with balsamic vinaigrette or lemon juice before serving.

7. Tuna Salad Stuffed Bell Peppers:

Ingredients:

- 1 can (5 oz) tuna, drained
- 2 tablespoons Greek yogurt or low-fat mayonnaise
- 1 tablespoon Dijon mustard
- Salt and pepper to taste
- 2 bell peppers, halved and seeds removed
- Optional: diced celery or pickles for crunch

Instructions:

- In a bowl, mix together tuna, Greek yogurt or mayonnaise, mustard, salt, and pepper.
- If desired, add diced celery or pickles.
- Stuff the mixture into the halved bell peppers and serve.

These lunch recipes are not only healthy and filling but also easy to prepare, making them perfect for busy days while following the DASH diet!

Dinner Recipes

Here are some delicious and nutritious dinner recipes that align with the DASH diet:

1. Baked Salmon with Asparagus:

Ingredients:

- 4 oz salmon fillet
- 1 cup asparagus, trimmed
- 1 tablespoon olive oil
- 1 lemon, sliced
- Salt and pepper to taste
- Fresh dill or parsley (optional)

Instructions:

- Preheat the oven to 400°F (200°C).
- Place the salmon and asparagus on a baking sheet. Drizzle with olive

oil and season with salt and pepper.

- Top the salmon with lemon slices.
- Bake for 15-20 minutes, until the salmon is cooked through and flakes easily.
- Garnish with fresh herbs if desired.

2. Chicken Stir-Fry with Vegetables:

Ingredients:

- 1 lb boneless, skinless chicken breast, sliced
- 2 cups mixed vegetables (bell peppers, broccoli, snap peas, carrots)
- 2 tablespoons low-sodium soy sauce
- 1 tablespoon olive oil
- 1 teaspoon ginger, minced (optional)

- Cooked brown rice or quinoa for serving

Instructions:

- Heat olive oil in a large skillet over medium-high heat.
- Add chicken slices and cook until browned and cooked through.
- Add mixed vegetables and ginger; stir-fry for about 5-7 minutes until vegetables are tender.
- Stir in soy sauce and cook for an additional 2 minutes.
- Serve over brown rice or quinoa.

3. Quinoa Stuffed Peppers:

Ingredients:

- 4 bell peppers, halved and seeds removed
- 1 cup cooked quinoa

- 1 can (15 oz) black beans, rinsed and drained
- 1 cup corn (fresh, frozen, or canned)
- 1 teaspoon cumin
- Salt and pepper to taste
- 1 cup salsa (optional)

Instructions:

- Preheat the oven to 375°F (190°C).
- In a large bowl, combine quinoa, black beans, corn, cumin, salt, and pepper.
- Stuff the mixture into the halved bell peppers and place them in a baking dish.
- Pour salsa over the stuffed peppers if desired.

- Cover with foil and bake for 30-35 minutes until the peppers are tender.

4. Vegetable and Bean Chili

Ingredients:

- 1 tablespoon olive oil
- 1 onion, chopped
- 2 cloves garlic, minced
- 1 bell pepper, diced
- 2 carrots, diced
- 1 can (15 oz) diced tomatoes
- 1 can (15 oz) kidney beans, rinsed and drained
- 1 can (15 oz) black beans, rinsed and drained
- 2 cups vegetable broth (low sodium)
- 1 tablespoon chili powder
- Salt and pepper to taste

Instructions:

- Heat olive oil in a large pot over medium heat. Sauté onion and garlic until soft.
- Add bell pepper and carrots; cook for another 5 minutes.
- Stir in diced tomatoes, kidney beans, black beans, vegetable broth, chili powder, salt, and pepper.
- Bring to a boil, then reduce heat and simmer for 20-30 minutes.
- Serve hot, garnished with fresh herbs if desired.

5. Grilled Chicken with Quinoa Salad

Ingredients:

- 1 lb boneless, skinless chicken breasts

- 1 cup cooked quinoa
- 1 cup cherry tomatoes, halved
- 1 cucumber, diced
- 1/4 cup red onion, diced
- 1 tablespoon olive oil
- Juice of 1 lemon
- Salt and pepper to taste

Instructions:

- Season chicken breasts with salt and pepper, and grill until cooked through (about 6-7 minutes per side).
- In a bowl, combine cooked quinoa, cherry tomatoes, cucumber, red onion, olive oil, lemon juice, salt, and pepper.
- Serve the grilled chicken alongside the quinoa salad.

6. Baked Sweet Potatoes with Black Bean Salsa

Ingredients:

- 2 medium sweet potatoes
- 1 can (15 oz) black beans, rinsed and drained
- 1 cup corn (fresh, frozen, or canned)
- 1/2 cup diced red onion
- Juice of 1 lime
- Salt and pepper to taste
- Fresh cilantro for garnish (optional)

Instructions:

- Preheat the oven to 400°F (200°C). Pierce sweet potatoes with a fork and bake for 45-60 minutes until tender.

- In a bowl, combine black beans, corn, red onion, lime juice, salt, and pepper.
- Once sweet potatoes are cooked, slice them open and top with black bean salsa.
- Garnish with fresh cilantro if desired.

7. Zucchini Noodles with Marinara Sauce

Ingredients:

- 2 medium zucchinis, spiralized
- 1 cup marinara sauce (low sodium)
- 1 tablespoon olive oil
- 2 cloves garlic, minced
- Salt and pepper to taste
- Grated Parmesan cheese (optional)

Instructions:

- In a skillet, heat olive oil over medium heat and sauté garlic until fragrant.
- Add spiralized zucchini and cook for 3-5 minutes until tender.
- Stir in marinara sauce and heat through.
- Season with salt and pepper, and serve topped with grated Parmesan if desired.

These dinner recipes are balanced, flavorful, and easy to prepare, making them perfect for a healthy meal following the DASH diet!

Snacks And Desserts

Here are some healthy snacks and dessert ideas that align with the DASH diet:

Snacks

Veggies and Hummus:

- **Ingredients**: Carrot sticks, cucumber slices, bell pepper strips, and hummus.
- **Instructions**: Slice the vegetables and serve with a small bowl of hummus for dipping.

Greek Yogurt with Honey and Nuts:

- **Ingredients**: 1 cup low-fat Greek yogurt, 1 tablespoon honey, a handful of nuts (like almonds or walnuts).

- **Instructions**: Top the yogurt with honey and nuts for a protein-rich snack.

Fruit and Nut Energy Bites:

- **Ingredients**: 1 cup oats, 1/2 cup nut butter, 1/4 cup honey, 1/2 cup chopped dried fruit (like apricots or dates), and 1/4 cup nuts.
- **Instructions**: Mix all ingredients in a bowl, roll into small balls, and refrigerate until firm.

Cottage Cheese with Pineapple:

- **Ingredients**: 1 cup low-fat cottage cheese, 1/2 cup pineapple chunks (fresh or canned in juice).
- **Instructions**: Combine cottage cheese and pineapple in a bowl for a sweet and savory snack.

Air-Popped Popcorn:

- **Ingredients**: 1/4 cup popcorn kernels.
- **Instructions**: Air-pop the popcorn and season lightly with salt or nutritional yeast for a cheesy flavor.

Desserts

Baked Apples:

- **Ingredients**: 2 apples, cored and sliced, 1 teaspoon cinnamon, and a drizzle of honey (optional).
- **Instructions**: Preheat the oven to 350°F (175°C). Arrange apple slices in a baking dish, sprinkle with cinnamon and honey, and bake for 20-25 minutes until tender.

Chia Seed Pudding:

- **Ingredients**: 1/4 cup chia seeds, 1 cup unsweetened almond milk, and 1 tablespoon honey or maple syrup (optional).
- **Instructions**: Mix chia seeds and almond milk in a bowl, sweeten if desired, and refrigerate for at least 4 hours or overnight until thickened. Top with fresh fruit before serving.

Frozen Yogurt Bark:

- **Ingredients**: 2 cups low-fat yogurt, 1/2 cup mixed berries, and a handful of nuts or seeds.
- **Instructions**: Spread yogurt evenly on a parchment-lined baking sheet, sprinkle with berries

and nuts, and freeze until solid. Break into pieces and enjoy!

Dark Chocolate Dipped Strawberries:

- **Ingredients**: 1 cup fresh strawberries and 1/2 cup dark chocolate (70% cocoa or higher).
- **Instructions**: Melt the dark chocolate in a microwave or double boiler. Dip each strawberry halfway into the chocolate, then place on a parchment-lined tray to cool.

Banana Oatmeal Cookies:

- **Ingredients**: 2 ripe bananas, mashed, and 1 cup rolled oats.
- **Instructions**: Preheat the oven to 350°F (175°C). Mix mashed bananas with oats, drop spoonfuls

onto a baking sheet, and bake for 10-12 minutes until set.

These snacks and desserts are not only satisfying but also nutritious, making them great choices while following the DASH diet!

CHAPTER FOUR

Cooking Techniques For Healthy Eating

Here are some healthy cooking techniques to incorporate into your meals, promoting better nutrition and flavor while aligning with the DASH diet principles:

1. Steaming:

- **Description**: Cooking food with steam helps retain nutrients and flavor.

- **Best For**: Vegetables, fish, and chicken.

- **Tip**: Use a steamer basket over boiling water or a microwave-safe steamer.

2. Baking:

- **Description**: A dry cooking method that uses an oven, reducing the need for added fats.
- **Best For**: Fish, chicken, vegetables, and whole grain casseroles.
- **Tip**: Use parchment paper or a non-stick baking spray to reduce sticking.

3. Grilling:

- **Description**: Cooking food over direct heat adds flavor without excessive fat.
- **Best For**: Meats, vegetables, and fruits (like peaches or pineapple).
- **Tip**: Marinate proteins to enhance flavor and tenderness while using less salt.

4. Sautéing:

- **Description**: Cooking food quickly in a small amount of oil over high heat.
- **Best For**: Vegetables, lean meats, and tofu.
- **Tip**: Use a non-stick skillet or a small amount of healthy oil (like olive oil) to keep calories in check.

5. Roasting:

- **Description**: Cooking food in the oven at high heat allows for caramelization and flavor development.
- **Best For**: Root vegetables, chicken, and fish.
- **Tip**: Toss vegetables in herbs and spices instead of oil to enhance

flavor without adding extra calories.

6. Slow Cooking:

- **Description**: Cooking food slowly at low temperatures allows flavors to develop.
- **Best For**: Soups, stews, and whole grains.
- **Tip**: Use lean cuts of meat and plenty of vegetables to make hearty meals.

7. Blanching:

- **Description**: Quickly boiling food and then plunging it into ice water to preserve color and nutrients.
- **Best For**: Vegetables like green beans, broccoli, and carrots.

- **Tip**: This technique can also help reduce bitterness in certain vegetables.

8. Pressure Cooking:

- **Description**: Cooking food quickly under high pressure retains moisture and nutrients.
- **Best For**: Beans, grains, and tougher cuts of meat.
- **Tip**: Always follow the manufacturer's instructions for safe use.

9. Stir-Frying:

- **Description**: Cooking small pieces of food quickly over high heat in a wok or skillet.
- **Best For**: Vegetables, chicken, tofu, and shrimp.

- **Tip**: Use minimal oil and add vegetables in stages for even cooking.

10. Fermenting:

- **Description**: Using bacteria or yeast to preserve food, which can enhance flavor and increase probiotics.
- **Best For**: Vegetables (like kimchi or sauerkraut) and yogurt.
- **Tip**: Experiment with different spices and vegetables to create unique flavors.

General Tips for Healthy Cooking:

- **Use Herbs and Spices**: Enhance flavor without adding salt.

- **Choose Whole Grains**: Opt for brown rice, quinoa, and whole grain pastas over refined grains.

- **Portion Control**: Use smaller plates and bowls to help manage serving sizes.

- **Limit Added Sugars and Fats**: Focus on whole foods and natural sweetness from fruits.

Incorporating these cooking techniques can help make healthy eating enjoyable and flavorful while supporting your overall health goals!

Eating Out On The DASH Diet

Eating out while following the DASH diet can be manageable with some planning and mindfulness. Here are tips to help you make healthy choices at restaurants:

1. Choose Wisely:

- **Opt for Grilled or Baked**: Look for dishes that are grilled, baked, or steamed rather than fried or breaded.
- **Select Lean Proteins**: Choose options like chicken, turkey, fish, or plant-based proteins like beans and tofu.

2. Control Portions:

- **Share Dishes**: Consider sharing an entrée or ordering smaller portions to avoid oversized servings.

- **Ask for Half Portions**: Many restaurants will accommodate requests for half-sized meals.

3. Load Up on Vegetables:

- **Choose Vegetable-Based Dishes**: Look for salads, stir-fries, or vegetable sides.

- **Request Extra Vegetables**: Ask for additional veggies in your dish or as a side.

4. Mind the Sauces and Dressings:

- **Ask for Dressings on the Side**: This allows you to control how much you use.

- **Opt for Vinegar or Lemon Juice**: Use these instead of creamy dressings or heavy sauces.

5. Limit Sodium:

- **Request Low-Sodium Options**: Ask if the chef can prepare your meal with less salt or seasoning.
- **Avoid Processed Foods**: Steer clear of dishes that might have high sodium ingredients, such as processed cheeses or cured meats.

6. Be Cautious with Bread and Carbs:

- **Skip the Bread Basket**: Avoid extra calories and sodium by skipping bread or asking for whole grain options.

- **Choose Whole Grains**: If available, select whole grain options for rice, pasta, or bread.

7. Be Mindful of Beverages:

- **Limit Sugary Drinks**: Choose water, unsweetened iced tea, or sparkling water instead of sugary sodas.

- **Watch Alcohol Intake**: If you choose to drink, do so in moderation.

8. Satisfy Sweet Cravings Wisely:

- **Share Dessert**: Opt for a small dessert to share, or choose fruit or yogurt as a healthier option.

- **Skip the Extras**: Avoid desserts with heavy creams or syrups.

By making mindful choices and being aware of portion sizes and ingredients, you can enjoy dining out while staying true to the DASH diet principles!

Here are some strategies for overcoming challenges when following the DASH diet:

1. Meal Planning and Preparation

- **Plan Ahead**: Dedicate time each week to plan meals and snacks. This can help you make healthier choices and avoid last-minute fast food.

- **Prep Ingredients**: Chop vegetables, cook grains, and portion snacks in advance to make healthy eating more convenient.

2. Dining Out:

- **Research Restaurants**: Look at menus online before going out. Choose places that offer healthy options or allow for modifications.

- **Communicate Your Needs**: Don't hesitate to ask for changes, like low-sodium options or dressing on the side.

3. Social Situations:

- **Bring a Dish**: If attending a potluck or gathering, bring a DASH-friendly dish to share.

- **Focus on the Company**: Shift the focus from food to socializing. Engage in conversations and activities that don't revolve around eating.

4. Cravings and Temptations:

- **Identify Triggers**: Recognize situations or emotions that lead to unhealthy eating. Develop alternative strategies, such as going for a walk or drinking water.

- **Healthy Alternatives**: Stock up on healthier snacks to satisfy cravings, like fruits, nuts, or yogurt.

5. Staying Motivated:

- **Set Realistic Goals**: Break down your goals into achievable steps. Celebrate small victories to stay motivated.

- **Track Progress**: Keep a journal of your meals, feelings, and progress. This can help you stay accountable and identify patterns.

6. Managing Time Constraints:

- **Quick Recipes**: Find simple, quick recipes that can be prepared in under 30 minutes.
- **Batch Cooking**: Prepare larger quantities of meals to have leftovers for busy days.

7. Budgeting:

- **Plan Budget-Friendly Meals**: Focus on whole foods, legumes, and seasonal produce, which can be more affordable.
- **Buy in Bulk**: Purchase staples like grains, beans, and frozen vegetables in bulk to save money.

8. Dealing with Setbacks:

- **Practice Self-Compassion**: Understand that setbacks happen. Instead of feeling guilty, reflect on what you can learn and get back on track.

- **Stay Flexible**: Adapt your plan as needed. If you face obstacles, be willing to adjust your approach without feeling discouraged.

By implementing these strategies, you can navigate the challenges of the DASH diet more effectively, leading to a healthier lifestyle over time.

Integrating Exercise With The DASH Diet

Integrating exercise with the DASH diet can enhance your overall health and support your goals for managing blood pressure and maintaining a healthy weight. Here are some tips on how to effectively combine the two:

1. Set Realistic Goals:

• **Combine Nutrition and Fitness Goals**: Set specific, achievable goals for both your diet and exercise routines, such as exercising for 30 minutes most days of the week and incorporating more fruits and vegetables into your meals.

2. Choose Enjoyable Activities:

• **Find What You Love**: Choose physical activities that you enjoy, whether it's walking, cycling, swimming, dancing, or group classes. This makes it easier to stay consistent.

• **Mix It Up**: Incorporate a variety of exercises (aerobic, strength training, flexibility) to keep things interesting and work different muscle groups.

3. Schedule Regular Workouts:

• **Create a Routine**: Schedule your workouts just like appointments to ensure you prioritize exercise.

• **Short Sessions Count**: If you're busy, remember that shorter, more frequent workouts can be effective. Even 10-15 minutes of activity can add up throughout the day.

4. Stay Hydrated:

• **Drink Water**: Staying hydrated is crucial, especially if you're increasing your activity level. Aim for water before, during, and after exercise.

• **Healthy Snacks**: Consider a small, healthy snack (like a piece of fruit or a handful of nuts) before a workout for extra energy.

5. Use Exercise to Enhance Your Diet:

• **Build Muscle**: Strength training helps build lean muscle, which can improve metabolism and aid in weight management.

• **Burn Calories**: Regular aerobic exercise can help create a calorie deficit, making it easier to maintain or lose weight while enjoying DASH-friendly foods.

6. Track Your Progress:

- **Monitor Your Activity**: Use a journal or fitness app to track your workouts and food intake. This can help you identify patterns and stay motivated.

- **Celebrate Achievements**: Recognize your progress in both diet and fitness. Celebrating small victories can boost motivation.

7. Listen to Your Body:

- **Rest and Recovery**: Allow time for rest and recovery to avoid burnout and injuries. This is especially important if you're starting a new exercise routine.

- **Modify as Needed**: Adapt your exercise routine based on how your body feels and your lifestyle changes.

By combining the DASH diet with regular physical activity, you can create a balanced approach to health that promotes cardiovascular wellness, weight management, and overall well-being.

Managing Other Health Conditions With The DASH Diet

The DASH diet is beneficial for managing various health conditions beyond hypertension. Here's how it can help with specific health issues:

1. Heart Disease:

- **Focus on Heart-Healthy Foods**: The DASH diet emphasizes fruits, vegetables, whole grains, and lean proteins, which support heart health by reducing cholesterol levels and improving overall cardiovascular function.

- **Limit Saturated Fats**: Choose healthy fats, such as those from nuts, seeds, and avocados, while minimizing saturated and trans fats.

2. Diabetes:

- **Blood Sugar Control**: The emphasis on whole grains and fiber-rich foods can help stabilize blood sugar levels.

- **Balanced Meals**: Focus on meals that combine carbohydrates with proteins and healthy fats to reduce glycemic spikes.

3. Kidney Disease:

- **Lower Sodium**: The DASH diet's low-sodium focus helps reduce blood pressure and strain on the kidneys.

- **Potassium and Phosphorus**: Consult with a healthcare provider to tailor potassium and phosphorus intake, as these may need to be monitored in advanced kidney disease.

4. Osteoporosis:

- **Calcium and Vitamin D**: Include calcium-rich foods (like fortified plant milks and leafy greens) and ensure adequate vitamin D intake for bone health.

- **Limit Salt**: High sodium intake can increase calcium loss through urine, so the DASH diet's low-sodium approach supports bone health.

5. Weight Management:

- **Portion Control**: The DASH diet encourages mindful eating and balanced portion sizes, making it effective for weight loss or maintenance.

- **Nutrient Density**: Focus on nutrient-dense foods that provide satiety without excessive calories.

6. Gastroesophageal Reflux Disease (GERD):

- **Avoid Trigger Foods**: While the DASH diet promotes many healthy foods, be mindful of individual triggers (like spicy foods, caffeine, and fatty meals) that may worsen GERD symptoms.

- **Balanced Meals**: Smaller, balanced meals can help prevent excessive stomach pressure.

7. Metabolic Syndrome:

- **Weight and Blood Sugar Management**: The DASH diet can help manage weight, improve insulin sensitivity, and lower triglycerides due to its emphasis on healthy eating patterns.
- **Regular Physical Activity**: Combine the DASH diet with regular exercise for improved overall health.

General Tips for Managing Health Conditions:

- **Consult Healthcare Providers**: Always consult with healthcare professionals or registered dietitians before making significant dietary changes, especially for managing specific health conditions.

- **Monitor Progress**: Keep track of symptoms and progress with regular check-ins with healthcare providers to adjust dietary plans as needed.

Individuals can effectively manage a variety of health conditions and promote overall wellness by utilizing the DASH diet as a foundation.

Conclusion

The DASH diet is a nutritious and adaptable eating regimen that is intended to enhance cardiovascular health and overall well-being. It provides a variety of advantages for a variety of demographics, including those who are coping with hypertension, diabetes, heart disease, and other conditions, due to its emphasis on whole foods, including fruits, vegetables, whole grains, lean proteins, and healthy lipids.

The DASH diet promotes the prevention of chronic diseases, weight management, and blood pressure control by emphasizing nutrient-dense foods, reducing sodium intake, and promoting balanced meals. Furthermore, it can be effortlessly customized to accommodate specific dietary requirements, including vegetarianism or veganism, and to accommodate a variety of age groups, including the elderly and infants.

The DASH diet necessitates the incorporation of regular physical activity, smart choices when dining out, and mindful meal planning. Individuals can adopt the DASH diet as a sustainable approach to healthful living, thereby improving their quality of life and physical health, with the assistance of commitment and flexibility.

THE END